the sin

GW00459157

2012 ana Beyona

"**the simple truth: 2012 and Beyond** provides a wonderful healing journey that encourages readers to shed their image of being helpless victims, and learn the truth of who they really are - Divine Beings inhabiting an earthly body.

Filled with great depth of understanding, Ocean WhiteHawk's informative and nurturing insights free the reader from self-sabotaging stories and emotions, so that they may create a life overflowing with love, peace and happiness."

- **Bruce H. Lipton**, PhD, best selling author of the *Biology of Belief: Unleashing the Power of Consciousness*, *Matter and Miracles* and co-author of *Spontaneous Evolution: Our Positive Future (And A Way To Get There From Here)*

Also by Ocean WhiteHawk

JuicyWoman – A Spiritual Guide to your Feminine Radiance

Available at bookshops or order online:

www.oceanwhitehawk.com

the simple truth

2012 and Beyond

Ocean WhiteHawk

Published by
juicyspirituality.com
United Kingdom

www.juicyspirituality.com

Greenpeace approved FSC certified paper carry FSC logo.

Printed and bound in Great Britain by Lavenham Press, Suffolk

A CIP catalogue record for this book is available from the British Library
ISBN 978-0-9562538-5-9

To the Divine Being in all.

May You finally walk this earth

undisguised.

Dearest Wendy,
Shine your light and
bless the world with
your Radiance!
Lot of Love,
Joan xx

Contents

How You Become this Living Truth

Why This Book Has Come Into Being

By Ocean WhiteHawk

Earlier this year, I had settled down to write my second book. It was going to be another one for my women-empowerment series. Since I first published *JuicyWoman – A Spiritual Guide to Your Feminine Radiance* in 2009 (a book that has come to be regarded as a manual for women, enabling them to wash away their self-doubts and shine their radiance) I decided that I was going to dedicate most of my time and love working in the feminine arena. Imagine my surprise when Divine

Upstairs (my affectionate name for Source) knocked on my consciousness and said I had to put that book on hold, and write this one first. The instructions were clear – I had only one month to get the job done! Nineteen days of writing to be exact.

I now understand the significance of timing for the birth of this book. We've run out of the Old Time – time of fear, time of victimisation, time of indulging in illusions that hold us back from what we really are: glorious Beings of Light. The major planetary shifts are in grand motion as the cogs and wheels of the Cosmos turn to precipitate the birth of this New Era, the era of Love. This message is not new, but the moment is Now, hence the urgency for this book.

It's your chance to step up your human game and make it a Divine Game. It's an invitation to merge with Spirit, and emerge as God Beings. It's co-partnership with Infinite Intelligence to bring Heaven to earth.

The realisation of your Spiritual Destiny is here. **You are the one you've been waiting for.** Namaste.

– Ocean WhiteHawk

8 Sept 2011

Truth - The Living Information

You are born with a mission to fulfil because your human story is about to change forever.

What Every Human Needs to Know

Regardless of what your life experiences may have been, regardless of what you have been told, the truth is, YOU ARE VERY DEARLY LOVED indeed. This timeless Truth goes back a very long way, beyond the existence of planets, galaxies and even star systems, never mind your birth in this lifetime.

But the moment you took this physical birth, you were sold a concept, one that was based on Self-forgetting, and suffered a profound disconnection with the Origin of your existence – Infinite Intelligence. We also fondly refer to this All-Knowing Intelligence as God.

As an exquisite Child of the Universe, you are not meant to struggle on this earth, just so you exist as a human being.

There is no written legacy that says life needs to be hard. It's only an unconscious mind that assumes it should be so.

You ARE loved beyond measure, but the mind caught in duality may not think so. Perhaps many a time you felt as if you were left out in the cold - forgotten - and had to fight your way through a minefield of disappointments and heartaches in order to live the day. 'Where was love then?' you might have asked. *Love was still present.* But Self-forgetfulness veiled this Blessing from your experience.

This is part of your pre-programmed human agenda. On a soul level, you gave permission to go through a period of your life with blindfolds on, so you wouldn't be aware of the extended Helping Hands that were reaching out to you. It was necessary that you understood what pain and separation from Source felt like, so when the time comes for you to awaken and offer your Gifts to humanity, your compassionate heart will enable you to flow forth the awesome Love that you are.

Believe in the grand Divine Design of life. You have a destiny to fulfil, not as a human being, but as an awakened Love Master.

You are born with a mission to fulfil, because our human story is about to change forever. We are right on the edge of a spiritual revolution! Never before, in the history of mankind as we know it, have we come this far as a collective race to make this quantum leap into our Divine Nature. On a cosmic level, all eyes are on the human nation right now. There is great excitement as people all over the world are stirring from their deep soul sleep, and one by one, two by two, four by four and so on, until thousands by thousands and millions by millions, we engage our breath-taking Power to flip our collective consciousness back into Spirit again.

Power Focus
Do yourself a loving favour and see that there is a greater reason to you being alive.

Power Statement
"There is a Higher Purpose to my life because I am in partnership with God."

Life is not the problem. Your spiritual amnesia is. Know thyself is the key to your ultimate freedom.

Wake Up, Sleeping Beauty!

The spell of soul sleep that we are under is a deep one for many. Soul sleep is when you have been hypnotised by the collective belief of the race to do with ill health, injustice, limitation and death. These are mortal thought-forms, confined within a lower band of energies which sap your innate Power to transmute negativity into life-enhancing energies.

Who are you, really? You are definitely not your name or the labels you've been given. You are not your past experiences either, although you may think they define you. And you are not your self-invented ideas of who you think you are, or your self-criticisms. All these fall under the general heading of 'Human Programming'!

And don't think that this programming shouldn't be so; that we should never need to go through what we did. Indeed, gems can be lovingly excavated from the gloomy caves of our trying past. Often, the more challenging the experience, the bigger the precious jewel there is. Through understanding, and assuming full responsibility for your soul choice to learn from that darkness, you are then able to untangle that particular life-choking knot, and release the creative energy into the flow of your life. To create what makes you happy.

You are the Creator, and you are the creation of your life. You create the distortions you see, and you create the wondrous miracles of joy and laughter. The uncomfortable bits are simply pressure points to make you stop the track you're on, apply your wisdom, and proceed again in a kinder direction. The exquisite ones are reminders of how dearly loved you are.

Everything you have experienced has been precisely engineered to bring you to this great moment for a beautiful and holy Purpose – to birth Light and Love into the dark corners of life. After all, the most effective way to bust a system is surely from the inside!

Life is not the problem, your spiritual amnesia is.

Forgetting that you are multidimensional, egoless, an all-powerful Entity, you waste much of your precious energies arguing with illusions. Illusions are nothing but the mirror image of your distorted thinking.

In Truth, in the larger all-encompassing Reality, you are still safely connected to the Divine Intelligence of which you're an intrinsic component. Wake up from your slumber! NOW! The joy and truth of what you are awaits you. Your power to heal and transform darkness, to be of sweet service to humanity, is before you.

Power Focus
Question the mundane so that the magnificence of what you are can be revealed to you.

Power Statement
"Powered by Infinite Intelligence, I AWAKE to see that everything belongs to me."

*Your true Life is infinitely larger,
and more expansive than the night sky
you gaze into on a starry night. Never for
one moment think you're insignificant.*

The Bigger Picture

When you finally direct your human focus away from the microscopic view of your 'imperfect' life, stand back, and take a deep breath. A big sense of soul relief will overcome you.

After all, you have been waiting all your life for this precious moment! When there is no going back to running round in circles, chasing after things that keep eluding you, like transient happiness, money, relationships, and outer success of any kind, you will be ready for what God has been trying to give to you all along – your *Divine Birthright* to health, wealth and supreme happiness!

Once you step back from indulging your precious attention in things that have gone 'wrong' in your past, you will lighten up. You will come to see that all events, including the so called negative ones, were only there with your soul's permission. On a higher level, you called them into being, to show you your misguided belief about yourself. It's simply a feedback mechanism you, as a soul incarnate, use to remind yourself to break out of the jail of limitation you have imposed upon your Divine Self.

Express a genuine desire to see the Truth of what your life is really about. In your quiet moments when you are alone with yourself, tenderly turn your face upwards towards infinite space, raise your hands and beseech God, *"What is REALLY the bigger picture of my life. What is my Greater Purpose? Tell me! Show me! I demand you answer me, God!!"* and don't stop until something happens. A day. A week. A month. No matter how long it takes, keep demanding until you get your clear, bright Answer.

Throw a tantrum if that's your style. Stamp your feet and pour all your juicy emotions and every ounce of precious energies into this Divine encounter. Wail and cry your eyes out. After all, people often cry, but how many actually cry for God? You'll be amazed how effective this technique is. Young children use it all the time to get their mother's attention!

Don't stop enquiring until the awesome Truth of your Divine Purpose is revealed to you. Once you know this wondrous Truth, you will be absolutely delighted that you have come to earth to play.

You have come to break through the illusion of death to be free from distrust and limitation. When you have mastered the fear of fear itself, the invisible platform you're standing on will steadily raise you up, so that the mass can benefit from your freedom.

Power Focus
Forget your human conditionings. Let them go as you would a piece of tattered garment. New golden robes are ready to adorn you when you claim your Worthy Self.

Power Statement
"I am a Love Master, here to carry out God's Agenda."

Engaging in the past is like having a ghost as your lover. The frolic will not make your skin tingle with delight and the kiss will be the kiss of death.

Living in the Past is the Kiss of Death

Living in the past is a violation of spiritual law. As these universal principles are immutable, contravening them will *always* cause you pain. It is designed to be so, to show you that going against the grain of your True Nature hurts. And it drains the colour out of your spirit too - enough to make you feel terribly bland and pale into insignificance at times!

We can safely say that living in the past is self-inflicted pain. On a soul level, it's your only way to get your attention, to stop you from proceeding down a Self-destructive route indefinitely. That would be a tragic waste of the Gift of who you are! The Universe loves you too much to stand by and watch you get submerged in this illusion without giving you instant feedback.

So we feel an 'ouch' and it gets our attention. Hopefully we are not daft enough to pop a pill into our mouth to numb this 'wake up' sensation and go back into soul sleep again.

What has gone is behind you. And yet it is such a bizarre human habit, to walk forward in life with one's head permanently fixed looking back over one's shoulder. Talk about giving yourself a chronic neck ache!

Human beings are the only species that keep regurgitating foul and toxic old stuff, and then re-consuming the unpleasant lot by re-living the disappointment and hurt! How insane is that? No animal of lesser intelligence on this planet would do that. That's what soul sleep does to you.

Life may have hurt you once, but you keep hurting yourself again and again by speaking about it. The event may be long gone, but each time you talk about it, you're tethered to the graveyard with tombstones and weeds as companions. That's not where the celebration of life is.

Gain your security from the wonders of the present, not from the disappointment of the past.

Living in the past is a method of failure. It steals your precious time and priceless energy. With no past to complain or even think about, a lot of your attention will be freed up. As a divine soul, you could channel the same life force to improve the human race instead. You'll feel better for it. Your vitality and passion for the present moment will return. From the zombie-like state, you'll come alive again!

Power Focus
The past belongs in the graveyard, so leave it there. It can't touch you anymore. If there is a happy story about it, do tell, as you'll be putting some sweet smelling flowers by the headstone. Otherwise, stay away. Not another word.

Power Statement
"I forgive my past, and I am grateful to know that I have God's Power to create a wondrous present and future for myself."

Your confusion is nothing but the mist that temporarily veils the intense rays of your shining Wisdom. Trust the Light will burn through any moment.

Human Confusion

Once you turn to seek the truth of your Identity, the old beliefs no longer serve. Let them fall away as leaves would on an autumn day. It is incredible how attached you can be to ideas that bind you to limitation. This is the bizarre behaviour of human beings, to say they want happiness and run blindly in the opposite direction. This chapter seeks to cast light upon some of the widespread human confusion that still shields you from your astonishing God Self.

Is stress part and parcel of being alive?
What is part and parcel of the human experience is fear. If your mind is incapable of self-doubt there will be no experience of stress ever plaguing you in your day or your restless nights. If truth is invited in, the powerful

Spirit of who you are *is* part and parcel of being alive. How comforting Truth is when you allow it.

Can I be spiritual and still have lots of money?
You can be spiritual and have anything you desire. It would make no sense for money to exist but not for you to have it. You are your own banker, and you decide when to give and when to withhold from yourself. What is in question here is not your spirituality but your self-worth. The moment you claim your Divinity is the moment you hit the jackpot.

How can I find time to pursue my spiritual journey when I'm so busy trying to make ends meet?
Turn this around and realise the reason you're so busy trying to make ends meet is because you don't know who you are. And what is spirituality but self-investigation to wake up from the illusion of who you are not? Be wise. Awakening to the God in you is your first priority. Everything else will unfold in the most miraculous manner that you couldn't imagine even in your wildest dreams.

Why can't I meet my true love when I have so much love to give?

Your first true love is the face that stares back at you when you look in the mirror. The foremost place that needs this bountiful love that you have saved for someone else is *within you*. Fall blissfully in love with the Spirit in you. The first union is *always* Self and Spirit. The outer beloved will show up thereafter. Love can never stay away from itself.

Why is death so undesirable, so frightening?

What is death but the continuation of life in a different garment? What is undesirable is not death itself, but your misunderstanding of what death is. What is so frightening about death is nothing but your belief in being annihilated from existence. It's not possible to obliterate Spirit. You live on regardless of your beliefs.

Power Focus

Question all forms of collective thinking. One by one, peel off the illusion to see your own shining Light.

Power Statement

"I now break away from the historical view of self."

Disengaging from the illusion of life frees you to experience the profound inner peace and exquisite bliss of what you truly are – God in a human body enjoying the delicious dance of Life.

The Schoolroom of Illusion

Do not give permanent reality to transitory things. This is the greatest cause of your human suffering.

As a divine soul, when you chose to dive into the dance of human existence, in that moment, you 'signed the contract' to enter into perceptual falsehood. In the wisdom of Eastern teachings, this is known as the Great Illusion. When you believe this illusion to be true, you will be fearful, embittered by the seeming injustice of life, and feel disempowered by things that are beyond your control.

Things are not what they appear to be. Beyond the smokescreen of human drama, the truth of why you have chosen to enter into a human life lies patiently to be revealed to you. When you understand this wondrous reason for your human birth, you will begin to see the perfection of the 'whys' in your life.

Why have you come? You have come to assume the role as a creator of the particular life you have chosen. To garner every experience as a blessed opportunity to awaken you to the truth of what you are – a joyous human God. You are not a lowly earthling, appealing to the help and mercy of a superior God. This would be as ridiculous as to say that the child is inferior to its mother.

Since your essential nature is God energy, which is Creation, you create. So, you've come to play with these creative energies, with the ignorance hat on at first, not seeing the direct connection between what you weave with thoughts and emotions, and the reality you find yourself in.

Self-responsibility is the theme of this Divine play from the moment you decide to incarnate, until the soul of who you are decides it's time to leave again.

You cleverly chose the childhood environment that was effective to bring into focus the precise human issues you have come to master. Abandonment, rejection, feeling unappreciated, ill-health, guilt, injustice, lack of self-worth, lack of wealth, lack of freedom - these are some of the distortions you have come to awaken from. To wake up is to break the illusion of their tyranny over you. In doing so, you graduate from this schoolroom of illusion, and resume the correct perspective of a creator, to see it all as a wondrous and valuable learning experience. And indeed, see everything as a blessing to return you to where your heart is.

In doing this for yourself, you will automatically be liberating the rest of human kind from the make-believe prisons they have locked themselves in.

Power Focus
Break out from this collective lie that you are at the mercy of some invisible force or God which decides what happens in your life. Claim your Creatorship now.

Power Statement
"I take responsibility for everything that happens, and I am now ready to create only good in my life."

Fear is nothing but an empty room.
How can an empty room hurt you?

Fear is the Greatest Illusion of All

Fear is a disbelief in yourself. It is the ultimate denial of your own Power. And in denying your own power, you unwittingly deny God's Power, because you are the divine offspring of this Infinite Intelligence.

To believe in fear is to affirm that something can be greater than the Omnipresent, the Omnipotent, the Omniscient. Can you see how fear doesn't make sense when you apply clear thinking to it?

When you give fear a podium to voice its dictate to you, it is like an angel folding her magnificent wings to hide under a toadstool because she believes she is safer there. *Fear can never make you safe.* It has no such ability, even though it speaks to you in tongues of safety and protection. *"Be afraid and I will keep you safe"* is the greatest lie.

Fear is a collective mind virus that breeds in the dark swampy grounds of ignorance. When you shine the light of your wisdom on it, it cannot withstand the fiery presence of Truth, and is obliterated from existence within your own doubting mind.

Where there is fear, there is no growth. Even fungus would not be able to flourish in such lifeless conditions, never mind you, a glorious Spirit who has come to earth to demonstrate your creative powers. Fret, worry, anxiety, apprehension, nervousness – all these are different guises of fear. You were never designed to spend so much time in this make-believe mind set. This creates all kinds of havoc in your body, and your life.

Fear is a vacuum, devoid of any sign of life and energy. So how can an empty space harm you? The next time you meet fear in the face, question its validity. You will find fear to be a nothingness that's trapped in an imagination that does not know its own goodness and power.

There is nothing to fear in the Universe, not even death, which is a necessity for the human vehicle that you've chosen to adopt in this lifetime. Out of your body, there is no death. After all, where would the butterfly be without the death of the caterpillar?

You fear when you doubt yourself. You fear when you separate yourself from your Source.

Fear does not exist. You invite this phantom in when you believe that something outside of you can have more authority and influence than your Inner Light – the God-force that makes up your Holy Self.

How do you dispel fear? *Through clear thinking. Through meditation. Through prayer.* Meet fear with open eyes and an open heart. Then switch on the fountain of courage. You will see that fear is just an empty room.

Power Focus
Knowing that fear is a falsehood that separates you from God, you do not avoid it. Instead, embrace fear into your Holy arms and transmute this poor little creature into Love.

Power Statement
"In the Divine Reality of who I am, fear does not exist."

You are the marvellous director of the holy pantomime of your life. See the funny side and things will look better.

Your Earthly Connections

In the infinite wisdom of your soul, you chose precisely the folks you deemed appropriate to be your parents. From their genetic make-up, to the kind of people they are, each facet was accurately considered before you made your loving choice. This is to ensure that they provide you with the necessary conditioning that will allow you to master what you're here to learn.

Know that no matter how it may look to the human perspective, every experience is valid – even those that seem negative.

From the viewpoint of souls, there are no victims, only agreed contracts to serve one another in the name of Love. Your spiritual growth and the expansion of your infinite nature remain the only agenda in God's benevolent eyes.

You will see that your so-called enemies are simply your soul buddies in disguise, loving you so much that they have agreed to play the 'bad guy', in order that you excel in your learning as a soul in a human vehicle. Most of all, they are here to help you master the powerful transformational tool of FORGIVENESS. Bless them for this tremendous gift. In doing so, your own heart will be free to dance with Love again.

Your family and friends, besides the gift of Love they bring, also have the important task of pressing your juicy buttons each time you get lost in the human drama. Whenever they frustrate you, it's only to remind you that you are arguing for limitations, having lapsed from your divine nature. On a soul level, they are here to give you instant feedback where you have forgotten who you are in the grand design of God's Reality: a gracious soul on a mission to come home to Love.

And your children, they are your teachers of tomorrow. Honour them, for their soul knows more freedom than you do. Most children now, especially those born to spiritually minded parents, come with advanced understanding about the nature of Reality. They are here to bring in new ways of being that are infinitely more loving and less fearful. Your job is to break down the old paradigm of fear so they can rebuild a better world, a more devotional and fear-free world, where Spirit presides over matter.

There is no such thing as a stranger either. Every soul who crosses your path is an angel who brings the immense gift of reminding you exactly where you have remembered, or forgotten, your True Self.

It is a masterpiece of soul planning, designing and structuring to engineer the precise people that are in your life!

Power Focus
Trust the wisdom of your soul that has chosen the specific actors in this human play of yours. Know that every single character bears a blessed gift.

Power Statement
"Everyone in my life is here to serve my highest good."

You are eternally loved. As Light Beings in a human body, you have more friends than those of the earthly nature. Rejoice.

The Realm of Spirit is Always on Your Side

Not a single soul on this planet exists without at least one spirit Guide to walk with them on their soul path.

You are *always* guided. But it is your human expectation of being on your own, adamant in your perception of aloneness, which obscures the loving presence of these wondrous Guides from your awareness. Eyes cast down and heart laden with low vibration emotions, your communication with the subtler realms of Spirit shuts down. Yet all you need to do is open your heart and call out in earnestness, and a loving Hand will extend itself to you.

Who are these Guides? They are the loving extensions of God, just like you are. They too are on the same divine path to their realisation of Godhood, just like you are. The difference between you and these Guides is that they are not under the spell of matter and illusion.

They too have a body like you, not of a dense material but of a higher etheric substance. You also have an etheric body. In fact, it's what you use when you pop out of your body every night when sleep takes over. You as divine consciousness do not sleep. One simply vacates the bodily garment while repair and general housekeeping takes place, to ensure all organs function at their optimum level, ready to serve your blessed spirit again the next day.

Guides are the holy links between your human longing, and the truth of God. It is for this blessed reason that they are in your life. Their task is to assure you that you are forever loved and watched over. They guide your attention beyond the material, so that you come to see the wondrousness and creative power of your Spirit Self.

Your Spirit Guides are here to deepen your understanding of the non-physical reality, the non-linear dimension of who you are and what you have come to do in this lifetime.

Through Love, they teach and guide you into the higher ways of God, in order that you penetrate beyond this thin veil of illusion, and leave suffering behind. Their function is to shine the Light of Truth and Love into the dark corners of your misperceptions, thus liberating you from the imaginary bonds of erroneous thinking.

There is no solid division between you and these Light Beings. The idea of such separation is only in your mind. Be comforted that each time your heart voices its plea, it resounds through the whole Universe, and those on the Spiritual Planes, who have been assigned the sacred task of guiding you, are *instantly* by your side.

Power Focus

With worthiness in your heart, through meditation, prayer and a quiet mind, you will be able to work consciously with your Guides. Be open to receive.

Power Statement

"I am now ready to have clear communication with my Spirit Guides."

*Darkness and pain are only the ego's
resistance to the Love of who YOU ARE.*

Duality and Darkness

Darkness is not an existence by itself. It simply denotes the absence of light. In itself, it has no power to make you afraid. How can a shadow on the wall hurt you, an infinite Being of Light? Such is the lie of the mind. It is merely playing a game with you as you dwell in your Self-forgetting. From the viewpoint of Spirit, it would be like children in a brightly lit room, who close their eyes and say they are afraid of the dark.

Are you aware that you have the capacity to shine brighter than a million suns put together? What do you think your cells are made of? Each gorgeous cell is made of the light of Consciousness. And you have fifty trillion of them! The reason you are not blinding us with your Divine Radiance is because you have a belief that you are something else – a mortal trapped in a finite mind.

Because your consciousness is powerful, your mistaken belief acts as a dimmer switch, turning up the resistance (to God's Truth) and reducing the outflow of your divine current, thereby dimming your intense God Light. The more mistaken beliefs you have about your true nature, the less expression of your Light (joy, happiness, inner peace, compassion and love) is seen.

Darkness, evil and pain came into existence in your paradigm the moment your human mind took on the notion of separation from God. This created what you experienced as the Great Split from Oneness, the Source of all that is, and gave rise to imaginary concepts such as duality.

When you use your truth-seeing eye, and peer beyond the appearance of mind stories, you will see that Reality simply *is*. Beyond the judgement of 'good' and 'bad', everything simply is. When you adopt this true way of seeing, you will have no resistance towards things you cannot change. Pain will cease immediately for you.

Another name for darkness is ignorance. And what is ignorance but the lack of understanding. Spiritual Knowledge would be the perfect medicine for such an ailment. Everything is here to serve Light and Love. Your wondrous soul knows this. Only the personality thinks there is a different agenda and indulges in the imagination of fear.

Evil is the ignorance of God's Will and God's Law. It is Good obscured from its own bright nature. It is Love believing it is hate.

Your belief in such distortions weaves them into your experience. When you have worked through the maze of your misperceptions, you will come to see that *all is good.* You will finally relax into the infinite Light of who you are, and begin to spread your delicious radiance, dazzling others as you go along.

Power Focus

Train your eye to see that God is everywhere and in everything, even the darkest corner. Your safety lies in this holy perspective.

Power Statement

"I relax and know that wherever I am, I am still in the bosom of the Divine."

To know Infinite Source, you have to find out who you are beyond your human shell.

Love, Light and God

You and God are inseparable.

The Fall that religion sometimes portrays is only in the ego's mind. The truth is you have never left the Garden. You have never been away from the Divine. The fruits of joy and plenty are still on the trees waiting for you. The only damnation, if ever there was one, is a belief invented by the human mind, not God.

Your consciousness is made of divine substance. Not that your mind can understand it, as it has no understanding in the non-linear domain.

Your nucleus is of God, so you don't need to do anything to deserve it. You simply are *it*. And no matter how much you disbelieve, or try to disown this divine identity, you remain a precious part of something Loving, Supreme and All-Powerful. That's the good news.

The not-so-good news is how quickly you move away from your True Identity when the external doesn't meet your approval. How hastily you grab the guise of a victim and negate your power to grow and learn as a soul. How quickly you choose to forget that self-responsibility is the strength of your Spirit.

What is Light? It is *you* when you are at ease with yourself. Too often you obscure your brightness when you think you should be something else.

You shine when you are fulfilled by the moment.

What is Light? It is *you* when your love is not torn by the appearance of duality: the good and the bad, the right and the wrong. These are simply judgements of your finite mind. The luminosity of your consciousness is most dazzling when you can see the perfection that exists beneath the surface of disarray and chaos. When you can see that all movements of life are lovingly held in the mighty folds of Divine Love, you have broken the spell of illusion.

What is Love? It is *you* when you can see the flicker of light in a heart that is yet to open and in its self-forgetful state, causes injury and hurt to people you love.

What is Love? It is *you* when you forgive the seemingly unforgivable, because you know there is no place that your Love cannot enter.

What is God? Indeed it is more accurate to ask, "What is *not* God?". God is. And God is *you* when you step forward without any guilt, regret or fear in your heart. You will have finally pieced back your mind, heart, soul and body from their believed fragmentation. Life then awaits you to bless its bowed head.

Light is YOU.
Love is YOU.
God is YOU.

Power Focus
See your every moment as a sweet journey to waking up to the Light, Love and God in your cells and DNA.

Power Statement
"I am now ready to let the awareness of my God-Self into my life."

You are God in human form,
experiencing the delights of Matter.

Your God Evolution Story

In the beginning, there was only Sublime Stillness that was You. There were no galaxies, no stars, no planets. No other life-forms. Nothing, but You. You were known by a different name then: Oneness, God, Infinite Intelligence. Your Cosmic Awareness filled the endless unbounded space and eternity. You were everywhere. You were all there was, and you felt unmet and un-experienced because there was nothing outside to look in.

So You decided to have an adventure into movement, and that was when the dance of Life began. You lovingly split Yourself in two, and Duality, the Dance of Polarity was born. From You came forth the Divine Masculine and the Divine Feminine, both equal in their creative power and at the same time, complementing the other. It was clever how You designed that each contained the other within. This was the beginning of your Divine Expression as Love.

This Cosmic Adventure gained momentum and You began to explode into myriads of life-forms, having such fun and joy, no longer alone in Your Existence. It was ingenious how each of these individualised aspects of You still contained the entire blueprint of your Divinity – a marvellous design indeed! Even inanimate objects bore your Divine Stamp.

The day came when You decided to inhabit matter. To squeeze your expansive Self into such density was no comfy wear. It was like wearing shoes one size too small on a permanent basis! But the game of Life was so enticing, so rich in its constant shifting kaleidoscope of colours, sounds, and textures, as well as emotions, ideas and dreams when You took the form of sentient beings.

God became human. Many unspoken aeons have passed since. It is so long ago that you can barely remember being an angel, never mind a God.

Many of you no longer have a conscious link with your other multidimensional selves. Firmly rooted in the spell of matter with all its human conditionings, you have forgotten that you have come to give perfect expression of the God You Are. Heavily polarised in the thinking mind and dense human emotions, you have inadvertently adopted human ways at the expense of your Divine Identity. In doing so, the balance of Life is lost and neither Spirit nor matter stands to gain from this Venture.

Humans are now right at the precipice of this holy remembering. The time has come to awaken this Spiritual Giant within. A new Earth is beckoning.

Power Focus

Begin to wean yourself away from the collective ancestral human ways and see yourself as a beautiful integral part of this Universal Intelligence.

Power Statement

"I am more than human. I am Divine in essence."

In a bizarre sort of way, you have come to learn what you are not, in order to be what you really are.

Your Human Costume

What is familiar does not mean it's true. Because you are accustomed to seeing your biological structure, you assume you're a body. The body is only your temporary vehicle to navigate through this earthly realm. It's a beautiful design of nature, composed of earth, water, air and fire. It has its own innate intelligence and other than providing it with the right fuel (appropriate solids and liquids!) it pretty much regulates itself without a lot of input from you. It even heals itself when you get out of the way! What a marvellous instrument it is! But it's definitely not who you are. Far from being a biological marvel, you are pure Spirit. Your soul is but an individualised aspect of God.

When the God Particle of who you are decided to become human, all aspects of the soul's needs and desires were profoundly studied. The right DNA, sex, race, culture, time frame, biological family, location and time of birth, and your physical, mental and emotional capabilities, were sorted out. Everything meticulously sorted out and nothing left to chance.

The most suitable connections are then made with soul groups like yourself, who are incarnated to provide you with the exact openings you need to awaken your consciousness back into Light.

You have taken this human personification many, many times before. At each precious birth, you have come to master a specific syllabus in the curriculum of the human schoolroom. Subjects range from *rejection, abandonment, betrayal, injustice, lack, and disempowerment to love and forgiveness.* Each time you graduate from a particular lesson, you move on to the next, but with more soul power at your disposal.

Through each human life, your learning gathers momentum until it reaches a critical point where your soul begins to wise up. Your spiritual eye opens and you begin to see the bigger picture of your existence. You begin to feel that you no longer fit into the normal agenda of human living and survival. Your soul feels restless inside. It no longer satisfies you to just eat, drink and be merry. You are ready for something greater, more wondrous than the human dream. It's the Divine Vision that you have come for this time.

Power Focus
Be at peace with everyone and everything that is in your life. See all are in service of your wondrous awakening.

Power Statement
"I bless everyone and everything in my life for their generous gifts to me."

Happiness is God's Truth.
Happiness is your natural state
when you don't believe what your
unkind mind says.

God's Will for You is Perfect Happiness

God wants what you want for you. God wants what makes you smile. If God has an agenda, it would be this – for you to live happily ever after. *Forever.*

God's Will for you is pure happiness. Whatever your blessed heart desires, you can have. If you find this hard to believe, it's not because it's not true. It's because you have donned the human garment for so long, that you have turned towards the outside for the riches that your heart seeks: mental, emotional, physical or spiritual. But there you will never find what can only be found on the inside.

You can have perfect health if you so wish. It would mean taking time to understand how this biological mechanism works and support its function by giving it the right kind of fuel and physical discipline that encourages the flow of life-force it needs to heal and regenerate itself. It also means getting control of your worry thinking patterns, so you don't put the natural system under duress and strain.

Abundance, not scarcity, is the truth of life. God is your Supply, so why wouldn't this Divine Intelligence want you to have whatever you need *and more*? Why would this All-Knowing Source bestow more to others and not to you? The root cause lies within. It's your *belief in lack* that blocks your awareness to this Divine Bounty. You believe in lack because you think you have to provide everything for yourself. And as you experience yourself as a finite being with limited capabilities, life becomes a worrying experience! You learnt this limiting human view from those around you. But when you invest your faith in Spirit rather than in matter, you can be sure that everything your soul needs will be amply provided for.

Everything your blessed heart wants is already given to you. You only need to be bold and claim it as your birthright to have. This includes Love, sweet Love.

Love is what you are. But as long as you're looking for it externally, you will not see it, not even when Love is staring you in the face. You will become aware of its sweet Presence when have forgiven yourself completely and utterly. It's your unkind judgement of yourself that veils you from experiencing Love in every waking moment.

Power Focus
Be willing to embrace a new truth that you are here to be a happy Spirit in a human body! And refuse to surrender your happiness just because the outside doesn't match with your thinking.

Power Statement
"I am the authority of my happiness. Nothing can take it away without my permission."

*Beyond the confines of form
and matter, your Awareness touches
all corners of the Universe.*

The Descent from Awareness

As a God Particle, you took the great cosmic adventure of splitting yourself up, filling all corners of the Universe with your Divine Essence. But wherever you were, you knew of your True Identity. Each time you took on a different form to give expression of your Perfect Self, when the purpose of creation and enjoyment was over, you would relinquish this temporary sheath and merge back into the Oneness again until the next outward bound creative adventure. This way, the full awareness of your Divinity was always maintained.

Associating with matter only when you chose to, you kept your original sense of Spirit Self intact, all the while remaining whole, pure, holy and connected with the pervading Infinite Intelligence. You only acquired the material clothing of your Spirit for the purpose of creation and enjoyment but never once forgetting who you were, never confusing the body to be the essence and power of life.

However, as you drove deeper into matter, these individualised aspects of you started to identify more and more with form and matter. A fondness towards the beauty of form and structure began to grow in your luminous awareness. And with it, a more intense sense of self as a separate entity from Source developed. Eventually, instead of surrendering the temporal form, your attachment towards your individuality took over. The ever more tangible and beautiful covering of shimmering individuality captured your attention and you chose to stay on. You stopped coming Home to the ocean of Divine Loving where you would be recharged and renewed, ready to personify Perfect Love again.

This was the beginning of your fall from the greater awareness of your Divine Lineage. As you took on the dense human form and became lost in the distractions of its five senses, you began to close your all-seeing eye and retract the delicate etheric antennae within your spiritual body used for higher communication. Conscious links with the infinite ocean of All-Knowing Intelligence became weak and eventually, non-existent.

When you define yourself without regard to your source in the Timeless Presence out of which this universe expands, you keep repeating the historical culture and conditions of human nature instead of personifying your Divine Attributes to progress the race.

When you define yourself in isolation, your senses deceive you and blind you to the Higher Truths within. They lock you into a partial perception of the delightful Universe in which you live. Your creative Power becomes inaccessible to you through your limiting thought-forms. But the hour of awakening has come.

Power Focus

Open your inner eye and see Life infused with Spirit. Behind every appearance is a deeper purpose and meaning.

Power Statement

"I now choose to see Truth and become aware of the Greater Reality where my Spirit resides."

*When your only desire is to serve
God, your wish becomes the command
for the Universe.*

Your Will is God's Will

Your will is your resolve. It is your power to bring into creation whatever your mind fancies. Once you lock your focus onto a goal you desire, the direct application of your will translates into an action plan. The implementation of this action plan over a period of time, depending on how considerable your goal is, invariably brings you the results you're looking for.

Your will is stronger than any physical manifestation. When applied in harmony with higher laws, all your aspirations become a living reality for you.

Being a Spirit encased in a human vehicle, due to the projected existence of a self-invented egoic mind, your will splits into two: the lower and the higher will. The lower will is personality driven, busy driving your attention and energy to achieve outer things. It's a body based will. It functions in isolation from the power of Oneness. Its effectiveness fluctuates according to your emotional dictates. It's the will of the senses.

Your higher will, however, has a different purpose and is cosmically programmed to align to God's Will. When your life focus moves away from the preoccupation of lower instincts and survival, and you begin to live as a conscious Divine Being, your will and God's Will become one and the same.

The Will of Great Spirit is to evolve all sentient life back to its spiritual nature of Love, Light and Truth. Its sweet longing is to progress individualised souls like you, to finally come Home, not unlike the story of the prodigal son.

When you take the final step to move out of your personal identity into your collective Being, the potent power to transform the old restrictive and limiting human ways becomes yours. For what is God's Will but the unlimited Power to sweep away the debris of the old systems of fear, making way for the New, the path of Oneness and Love that is flooding into our energy fields as we speak?

Invoking your higher will means you have unwavering faith in the Infinite Intelligence that's behind all workings of life. Your will, when mixed with unreserved faith in God, becomes an immense column of Higher Power to awaken the consciousness of humankind. When you use the eye of faith, you can then bring into operation the higher spiritual laws. These blessed laws are here to ensure that you will always be safe and looked after while you serve humanity with your spiritual gifts and soul talents.

Power Focus
Have faith in God, faith in humanity, faith in all-Good and faith in yourself.

Power Statement
"God's Will is my will. All is being done with ease and joy."

*When you understand what you are,
you will know the Universe and its
enchantment.*

Freedom by Understanding

You will come to see that life is an astonishing existence when you realise that you are one great unlimited Whole. Living information from the cosmos will be at your disposal. On a personal level, there will be no lack or want. No hollow feeling or foreboding sense of emptiness, even when surrounded by outer possessions.

Spirit wants to help you to live a real life; a life of deep meaning; a life of purpose. After all, you *are* designed to be great. As a conscious soul, you are fully equipped to bring the essence of Spirit into full manifestation.

But how adamant the ego is to deny your remarkable God Nature! Its seductive persuasions about fear and lack are constantly whispered in your human ear.

This is because the ego is not in favour of your enlightenment. It does not believe in the certainty of God. It thrives on your artificial fear towards the Unknown. How do you stop yourself being conned by its tricks and insidious plans to keep you in your Self-forgetting? How do you find freedom in the midst of its woeful tales of threatened security and the uncertainty of your future?

By recognising what is true and what isn't.

The intellectual mind has no ability to distinguish between truth and falsehood. For example, if you happen to have the exciting experience of walking on a rope bridge suspended hundreds of feet in the air, do you notice how you cling on for dear life even though the bridge is perfectly secure and strong? How strange that you don't question its validity when the fearful mind speaks to you before you decide how you want to feel?

To find freedom from the bondage of the human quagmire, you must direct your gaze inward. Seek to understand the invisible workings of life. Read the appropriate books, on spirituality, on consciousness, on metaphysics. *"Seek and you shall find"* are words of truth. Invest time and energy in investigating the truth behind the appearance of all things. Summon your inner source of Wisdom. Enquire, enquire, enquire! Don't stop until Knowledge returns to your conscious mind.

Make Spirit the 'be all and end all' of everything you do. Focus on your soul development. Go on courses. Find a good teacher. Be in the company of people whose understanding is more advanced than yours. Let them enlighten you about the mysteries of the Universe. Meditate. Understanding the uncompromising Truths of the Universe will release you from dull human preoccupations and fear's tenacious grip.

Power Focus

Every morning and every night, expose your mind to spiritual teachings. The high frequencies behind the words will illuminate your consciousness, bringing clarity in your seeing.

Power Statement

"I am now ready to embrace the Truth of what I am."

Love is not selective like the mind.
It loves all and serves all.

The Ascent into Love

The choice for Love is why you are here this time round. It's a magnificent choice, a life extending choice, a holy choice.

Love is holy, because it has no concept of judgement, and it bars no one from its door. Love is pure, because it sees only innocence, even in the eyes of hate and evil.

Love is inexhaustible, because no matter how much Love you are able to soak up, from here to eternity, there is still plenty more where it comes from. And Love is the only currency that multiplies itself, and increases its quantity and value when given away: the more you give away the more you have.

There is nothing but Love. Matter is formed by Love. Atoms are bound by love. Your human frame is held together by Love. And where Love is absent, life begins to break down, for Love is the living information of Life. It gives living matter the reason to regenerate and repair itself.

Love is the common dialect of the heart, no matter the skin colour, age, sex, culture or heritage. Its non-verbal language brings down the unspoken barriers of the mind. Love extends invisible bridges across time and space, allowing consciousness to meet in Oneness with Beings, seen or unseen.

Love is maximal, so each time it gives of itself, it gives completely, keeping nothing back for itself. It is bold in its giving. Love is the highest frequency because Love is God in actuality, so each time you witness Love in action, know that you are gazing into the eternal face of the Divine!

Love performs miracles as well as being a Miracle.

Love is also what you are, but you are dimly aware of this astounding Truth. The fact that you walk around with the alms bowl for tiny scraps of affection and tenderness from the external world does not alter the truth that you are a Love Being in disguise.

The reason you are not aware of this heavenly bounty in you is because you have not allowed this magnanimous force into the parts of you which you have deemed unworthy. Beings of Utter Love are the ones who have forgiven themselves totally. Regrets. *Forgive.* Imperfections. *Forgive.* Mistakes. *Forgive.* Missed opportunities. *Forgive.* Forgive until there is nothing left to forgive. The perfect Love of who you are will stand unveiled. With no effort, your Love Presence will transform lives and ascend them into glorious heights.

Power Focus
Love cannot be taught nor practised, as Love simply is. You can however, practise the decision to Love. And it always begins with you.

Power Statement
"I love and accept myself, just as I am."

Illness is an outward manifestation
of inner turmoil
Spirit is the ultimate cure.

The Gift of Illness and Healing

The day will come when humans no longer need to manifest illness as a way of waking up from the delusion of matter, for what is illness but a call to come back to the truth and joy of Spirit. As this next Great Cycle of Cosmic Awareness continues to expand, understanding of your True Nature will increase ten thousand fold. Your consciousness will no longer be locked in matter, and you will have no need for ailments and disease as wake-up calls.

Every manifestation of illness has a gift in its loving hands. To receive the gift it brings, you need to first accept that there is a higher purpose for it to be in your body. Then listen deeply to that part of the body that's calling out for your Love. When you, as a blessed soul, truly pour the Love of who you are into that dis-eased part of you, spontaneous healing will take place. Miracles will happen. For what are miracles but the natural consequence of Love?

There is nothing to fear about an illness should it appear in your vicinity. The truth is, it is fear that has created the dis-ease in the first place, so to be afraid is to pour petrol into the fire in an attempt to douse out the flames!   But of course, a frightened mind would not know that it's only making matters worse, so during such intense times, let Love be the ultimate physician.

Can you love cancer should it be present in your body? Well, can you love a frightened child? Of course you can. You will sweep her up in your loving arms, administer your Love until fear vanishes from her eyes and spirit shines forth from them. That's how powerful your Love is.

Contrary to popular belief, it is not disease or illness that kills humans, but the absence of Love on a regular basis. Living in a culture that emphasises material success often causes the soul to negate self-Love. In the harsh pursuit of external success, self-neglect becomes a dangerous pattern. Following one's heart is no longer a priority, but producing results that measure one's worldly achievement is. And as the human system is not designed to live with a broken heart, ailments appear as an urgent call for self-Love.

As illness is the manifestation of a spiritual need, emotional confusion or mental commotion, it first exists in the non-physical realm of the auric field. The onslaught of trauma constricts the body and upsets the harmonious balance essential for health. But when attention is given in the form of deep questions to oneself, *"Why am I not happy?" "Am I living my true purpose?" "What is my passion?",* the route to healing will become obvious.

Sometimes, the blessed soul creates illness as a way to invoke the Healer within. *'Physician heal thyself'* are ancient words of wisdom, long-lost and forgotten in the quagmire of modern living. This gift of healing is now awakening in your cells as you read.

Power Focus
Remove all fears you have towards illness and disease, because they do not appear out of nowhere. Instead, infuse Love into your cells on a daily basis.

Power Statement
"Through Love, I take control of my health."

*Behind every wound is the profound
gift of Power and Spirit.*

Beyond the Language of Wounds

Since the emergence of counselling, therapy and support groups for every kind of emotional trauma, from child abuse and incest to domestic violence, our present day culture now has a proficiency in the language of wounds.

It is now common that the closeness and intimacy of a relationship is formed through the bonding of 'shared wounds'. Having gone through similar pains allows individuals to keep each other company in the world of their inflicted injury. In terms of support groups, what starts out as an intention to help people experience a nurturing and compassionate response to a personal crisis can turn into a dependency habit. Without a schedule for healing, one could become addicted to what we believe is support and compassion and become attached to the process of healing rather than being healed.

Notice how the ego loves repeating a story of victimisation. Unfortunately, talking about the pain you have gone through keeps you in the un-healed cycle. And that isn't the end of its mischief making either!

Do you use your wounds to control people emotionally by saying that their actions remind you of an old hurt you've experienced? Or do you let others use their wounds to control you? Observe how some people give themselves permission not to try, or give up their initial efforts of improving either their health or wellbeing, by dwelling on their past. It's an easier route for a disempowered personality to take.

The highest basis to begin healing is to acknowledge that you are more than just a human being. That you are Spirit temporarily rooted in matter, so you have the undeniable power of Source at your disposal to heal. This will allow you to have a strong backbone and believe in recovery as opposed to believing in being hindered by your predicament.

Healing is simple, but it requires dedication and commitment. Your first step is to identify the root cause of the pain. To do that, you need stop projecting your blame on the 'perpetrator' and turn inward to lovingly meet your wound face to face.

Never talk to someone about your wound if they have not transformed theirs, as they have no power to enable you to heal. Find a professional, or someone who has transcended their own wounds, to help you gain clarity on the real issue behind the wound.

Then identify the good that has come from it. Seeing the blessing behind the seeming misfortune becomes the healing agent that restores the peace in your heart. It aids the act of forgiveness, which is the most powerful spiritual tool we have in our psyche. Once healed, the only time you will speak of the wound story is to inspire others in their healing process.

Power Focus

Notice how repeating old stories of wounding cuts you off from your instincts of strength, and short circuits your connection to Spirit.

Power Statement

"I choose to see the blessing from hurtful experiences and be empowered by them."

The more you engage your spiritual brain to influence things around you, the more synchronicity, magic and miracles come your way.

Stepping into Your Right Brain

You belong to the New. You are people of the New Era. History is no longer pertinent to you as it was relevant to your great forefathers and foremothers. Contrary to common thought, there is nothing that you can learn from history, for the river of life surges swiftly forward and not backward. To assume that it is the fear of repeating the same mistakes of the past that has kept you safe and sane is an error. This interest and focalisation on out of date modalities have cost you your multidimensionality, and your ability to move your awareness in and out of the different planes of existence.

Your individualisation into matter and your spiritual amnesia have caused you to overuse your left brain, and under utilise your right brain.

Each brain hemisphere is unique in the specific types of information it processes. You don't just have one mind, but two. Hence there are times when you find yourself saying, *"I'm in two minds about this"*!

Your left brain is the home of your ego. It uses logic and reasoning to organise your thinking. It employs rules and regulations as an attempt to keep you safe in a little box, where fresh air, sunshine and spontaneity don't exist. This judging brain is highly competitive and constantly compares you with your contemporaries, noticing every little detail of what's not perfect, what's not right, what's not good enough according to its intellectual standards. When your consciousness is locked in this hemisphere, you struggle with time, especially with the past and the future.

Your right brain, however, is your spiritual brain. Your knowledge of your immortality and the eternal nature of your Being are accessed here. It is only capable of seeing the bigger picture and sees the intricate connection between everything and everyone. When your consciousness resides in this hemisphere, you will experience yourself as a being of Love, profoundly linked with all other beings, incarnate or discarnate in the same fabric of Life. Your compassion abounds because you have the intuitive ability to feel into another's experience. You are spontaneous, carefree and imaginative and have no fear, because there is trust in the intuitive guidance that flows easily to your conscious mind. This NOW brain allows you to experience the richness of this present moment, and etch it forever in your remembering. It also gives you unlimited access to multidimensional information and high frequencies that are coming through your inner space, as the vibration of this planet increases for a paradigm shift to Spirit.

Humans only use 10 percent of their brain, the intellectual aspect, while 90 percent of the right brain, their spiritual aspect, remains un-activated. Life remains a solemn affair while this advanced Love aspect of who you are remains untapped.

Power Focus
Step into your Love brain, the grateful, joyful and innocent hemisphere. Think, act and feel from this spiritual plane and the blessed soul of who you are will finally BE HERE NOW.

Power Statement
"I choose to be intuitively guided in everything I do."

You are pure Consciousness, here to magnify the beauty and wonder of the physical domains.

The Light of Your Consciousness

Your mind is an exquisite device, and much of its ability is yet to be discovered. And the best for humanity has yet to come. In many ways, the two are beautifully linked. As you advance your understanding of your soul design and the origin of you, your marvellous capabilities will unfold in front of your eyes and astound you with their ingenuity. Your ability to move and manipulate energies, to calm the storm of emotions and raise frequencies to pure Love and intense Joy, will be demonstrated. You will then apply your creative skills to engender a life filled with the luxury of laughter, of uninhibited Love and the contentment of Spirit wherever you are, and whoever you are with.

Be bold and acknowledge that all you think you know may not be the whole story. Be willing to be shown the good news that there is more than what humans have witnessed on their television sets or spread across their morning newspapers so far. Open your mind so that you can make room for what you have yet to know.

What is calling for your greater understanding is in fact already within you. When you dive into the deep well of your Being, what you will find is light – the brilliant, sparkling white light of your eternal consciousness. When your mind is still, quiet from the incessant human chatter, you experience this Light as awareness, experiencing from an observer's point of view rather than the doer of actions.

The Light of your Consciousness is all-powerful. It is your Divine Awareness present in a biological form.

Whatever you focus upon, there you would energise to life the belief, the thought, the idea, with this Higher Consciousness. If your physical eyes could see it, it would look like an intense beam of light emitting from your eyes and forehead to the subject of your focus. When you do this consistently over a period of time, you will hatch your ideas, plans and inspirations into physical manifestation from the field of pure potential, where all possibilities lie.

This creative power has been dormant in your human system until now. You have been using it, but rather unconsciously. As the spiritual energies begin to swim into the atmospheric layers of this planet, and penetrate into you, you will become more aware that you are indeed an outward manifestation of Spirit. And you shall enjoy your blessed role as a cosmic gardener, lovingly tending to the most picturesque planet in this star system!

Power Focus
Practice unlocking your attention from the superficial and mundane aspects of your day by moving your awareness into being the observer, rather than the doer.

Power Statement
"I am the Light of Consciousness dwelling in matter."

*You are heralding in the frequencies
of Love that angels of Light may
descend on earth.*

New Children of the Future

The next two decades will be the most intense and prolific period of change for the human civilisation. As the waves of Light and Truth sweep through the consciousness of the race, on an individual and collective level, you will witness the breakdown of the old thought structure. All fear frequencies will have to go, to make way for the Love frequencies that are flooding into your quantum field of Reality.

Agents of Light like you have been infiltrating into Earth's biosphere since the age of darkness. Each of you comes with a specific task to assist during this epoch of Great Change. As time goes on you will find that you meet more and more kindred spirits along your path, sharing the common mission of being Light Workers while you're going through the similar journey of awakening from the spell of matter.

As you see new colours emerging from your sky, and sense the changes humming in the air, you will notice the children of today too shine a different light. Indigo children, crystal children, star children, all of them direct descendants of unadulterated Spirit who have come through the stellar gateways to participate in this Great Shift.

The System-Busters are known as Indigo children as they radiate a vibrant indigo ray in their auric field. They arrive preserving a strong sense of who they are, and often come across as demanding and in-your-face. Crystal children are more sensitive and softly spoken, with an air of innocence and otherworldliness about them. They are the Peace-Makers of the new race. Star children have a strong resonance of the extra-terrestrial, and they come bringing new ways of communication, like telepathy, as the norm. Very often, they are able to maintain a strong multi-dimensional awareness of their stellar heritage.

Their destiny is to bring in the new frequencies that are needed in order to flip the orientation of human consciousness from materialism back to Spirit on a collective level. They interpret Reality as God-in-Matter. They have a big task ahead of them, and need your help to succeed in their holy mission.

To enable them to incarnate fully into matter as conscious Light Beings, you must not restrain them with rules and dogmas of the old. Give them the tools of your understanding, but do not tell them who they should be. Keep their spiritual nature alive in their conscious mind by exposing them to high frequencies of Love and Unity. Do not teach them about fear or separation. They flourish, and will remain confident to be who they are destined to be, when they are not forced to fit into a paradigm that is sustained by fear and limitation.

They have come here to do what you have not yet done. See their beauty and perfection. They are here because you have called them into your existence.

Power Focus
Your role is to help these new children to grow in a way that they do not forget who they are.

Power Statement
"I awaken my mind to see these new children and help them bring forth their gifts to humanity."

*The Second Coming of Christ is not in
the form of one man but in the hearts
of all humans.*

The Return of Christ Consciousness in You

For aeons you have been lovingly and carefully prepared by Love itself, for the dawning of this excellent age that is poised so elegantly at the doorway of its holy emergence right now. Every part of you is being deeply cleansed, anointed with the sacred scent of sweet frankincense, and a new garment of Light draped across your soul. Waves of pure excitement and joy constantly erupt in your Being, but much of it is unconscious at the moment. You are waiting at the threshold of eternal time, to step forth at the perfect blessed hour, to enhance the world with the blessing of who you really are.

Seeds have been sown into your flesh and bones for the day when the living Truth within your biology awakens from its deep slumber in material consciousness. This is the second coming your sacred scriptures speak of in history. For the one whose heart is able to rise above worldly disturbances, this distinct message is clearly heard, not from a historical viewpoint, but an eternal perspective. Much of this Seed was set within humankind then. It's vital that you do not allow the limitation of organised religion to close your mind from this timeless living information that is unfolding within your own consciousness and DNA now.

What is Christ Consciousness? It is the *complete awareness* of everything and everyone as manifestations of Love. The chair you're sitting on, the clothes you're wearing, the air you're breathing, even the book you're holding in your hand are nothing but the perfect form of intangible Love. And how does Christ Consciousness relate to all things and all interactions?

As glorious Love itself.
As blissful Love enjoying Love.
As self-forgetting Love calling to Love.
As compassionate Love responding to Love.

Your Christ Self is nothing but your Love Self. Everything that seemingly exists outside the perpetual envelope of this Love is nothing but a distortion caused by your finite mind, a human conditioned mind-set that saw itself outside the perimeters of Eternal Love. How can All-There-Is be away from anything, including itself? Look again with your knowing heart and you will see a proverbial lie, a collective propagation of falsehood amongst the forgetful ones. However, the blessed hour has arrived. Christ Consciousness shall reign in you, in humanity, as well as your sanctified Earth, regardless of what the fearful ego might think.

The next nine chapters will give you helpful information on how you can assist in this global process of mass awakening by first transforming your own consciousness and vehicle. For once you have liberated your own system from the shadows in your mind you will have the Power, Light, and Love to restore God's Reality on earth. *You do so by incarnating the most holy and highest in you.*

Power Focus
From now on, see yourself as Spirit residing in a biological system. Think, feel and act as Love would, and refuse to believe you are anything else.

Power Statement
"I AM the holy Spirit and the holy flesh of God."

How You Become this Living Truth

Your body is the house for your living
Light. Be kind to it. Bless it and reside
in it with Joy.

Your Body –A Clear Vessel to House Love

Earth is a sensuous Universe in which the Spirit of who you are has come to play. The Divine motive to descend into the realm of the physical is for pure enjoyment and the celebration of life. After all, why do birds sing with such elation? Why do dolphins leap with such joy? Why do children play from dawn to dusk? It is to share God's great passion for life itself.

Your biological self is not designed to be lost in the world of doing, but to *enjoy* being alive in this space time continuum that the soul of who you are has chosen to visit at this eternal moment. The ways of old, the anxiety for modern survival, has riddled your body with low frequencies of judgement, fear and non-love. The manifestation of illness, heaviness and stiffness in your human frame reflects your Self-forgetting.

You are not your body, but indeed your body is the holy container in which you, Infinite Spirit, can give perfect expression of your Love. As such, you must now, in your infinite grace, raise the vibration of your physical vehicle to connect with the high octaves of your soul energies.

Drink plenty of water, for it is the healing water of life. Your fields need irrigation before they can provide you with the harvest of plenty. In the same way your body needs this life-enhancing fluid to wash out its wounds and lacerations from the daily affliction of an unenlightened life.

Eat with lightness and joy. Before you begin to partake of your daily food, close your eyes and take a precious moment to connect with Spirit. Use the focus to bring Peace into the hearts of humanity. See within your inner eye the downpour of Supreme Light, casting away the shadows of fear, greed and separation. Then proceed to enjoy your food. Let every mouthful be of gratitude for the life forms that gave of themselves in order that you live.

Give to the body the exercise it needs so that the physical heart may pump passionate and strong. Oil its joints with fluid movements so that calcification of rigid thinking can be removed. Dance to enhance its circulation. Rest when you hear its weary sighs.

Expose it to sounds and music that do not grate upon its natural rhythms and cycles. Mantras are high vibrational sounds that contain the power of Spirit. They are gifts from the cosmos to help you tune the physical body to the beautiful resonance of soul frequencies. Use them.

Before you vacate your body at night, lay it to rest with thoughts of regeneration and rejuvenation. When you awake to the inviting dawn, affirm how well and happily your physical vehicle will serve your Light for the new day. *Never criticise it.* Be grateful for it instead. Treat it with Love. It will serve your holy Purpose well.

Power Focus
Regard your body as a sensuous channel for you to enjoy the sounds, colours and textures of this physical universe. It is a divine vessel to house Love.

Power Statement
"I love and honour this body for hosting my Spirit."

*The polarity of your emotions shifts
from fear to Love the moment you
remember you are Spirit.*

Your Emotions – To Amplify Truth

In the blueprint of your human design, your emotions are meant to be molecules of your pleasure, your delight, your fiery passion and your happiness. Your quality as pure Spirit is unadulterated joy. Each particle of emotion in your biological system is made to sing with divine ecstasy when intoxicated with the devotion of Spirit.

Every emotion is the energetic raiment of your state of consciousness. They broadcast the thoughts in your mind to the outside world in vivid colours and hues of aliveness and enthusiasm, or dull shades of boredom and monotony. These energetic tones are not seen by the physical lens, but nevertheless are felt by the sensitivity of the soul.

Why do you feel the way you feel? Your emotions are primarily governed by your mind. They are experienced as a clear limpid pool when your mind is at peace with itself. Or as a tempestuous storm when your perception tells you that someone is taking advantage of you. The whole spectrum of emotions can vary from great stillness to utter rage or hatred depending on how your mind is translating the interface with another.

These dynamic energy movements have a regenerative or destructive attribute. They calibrate at different frequencies. The lower the vibration, the more destructive the force is against your own body and others around you. Emotions such as jealousy, sadness, resentment, anger, anxiety, fear and hate form a psychic shield that block the receptivity of living information that is constantly being transmitted to your Soul Essence. Over a period of time this causes the body to fall sick.

However, positive emotions like joy, love, peace, compassion and tenderness have life-enhancing qualities because they vibrate at high frequencies. These light frequencies keep you connected to the higher thoughts, visions and motivational currents of your Universal Being. The constant experience of such high calibrations has a spontaneous healing effect on your biology.

Your emotions are meant to amplify the truth of who you are. They broadcast to the external how you're seeing yourself in that crucial moment of interaction – a powerful entity of Spirit, or a disempowered human being. They are one hundred percent indicative of your thought patterns.

As a spiritual being, it is vital for you to master the ability to transform your lower emotions into higher forces of Love. When you feel upset, watch comedies. Laugh. You will feel better instantly. Qi Gong and breathwork are also effective in shifting emotional patterns. But the most powerful technique that you, as a Divine Soul, have is to change the thought that's causing the ripple of destruction. Train your mind to produce waves of delight and inner happiness at will, by focussing on thoughts of Love and Forgiveness. Before long, spontaneous joy will arise out of you, to honour the beauty and enchantment of Creation. And your emotions will broadcast that to the world.

Power Focus
Monitor your emotions and observe how they impact on your health and wellbeing.

Power Statement
"I have control over my emotions."

The mind that serves Spirit draws
the holy out of the unclean.

Your Mind – The Servant of Spirit

Your true mind is the Mind of God. It is one and the same. Tune out all outer influences, the crackling static noise of the fear-based projections of humans. You will quickly become receptive to the beautiful and sanctified thoughts of your indwelling Spirit. This is your True Identity. It is your conscious link to the Universal Intelligence that sustains your soul. It knows the exact path you need to take to fulfil your Divine Destiny.

Mind is the most powerful mechanism in your human system. The thoughts it churns out are the creative building blocks and cement that build your life the way it is. You are indeed the architect of your blessing or demise. The outcome of every happening and challenge is in your hands.

Mind turned outward becomes the slave of the ego. The dictates of such a mind are laced with poison. Judgement, criticism, fear and separation are some of its lethal prescription. In such instances, the mind becomes the seat of pain. It invents divisions between humans. It believes it can be happy at the expense of another. Such a mind is easily threatened, even by suggestions of shadow and the unreal! You are familiar with the afflictions of such a mind.

Mind turned inward into the infinite possibilities of Spirit is a Divine Mind, the Mind of Christ. This mind has no limitation; hence it is not cursed by wild imaginings of lack or non-safety. Such a mind has every creative tool and Spiritual Hand at its disposal to do what it wills, for such minds create kingdoms of genuine happiness and freedom for those blessed souls who have the good fortune to come across its path. Such illumed minds will always have Sublime Peace and Power to create benevolence for the human tribe.

A mind that is untrained is a dangerous mind. Like a car with a senseless driver, it creates carnage for the poor soul who has trusted the intellect, which has no Divine Knowledge, to navigate safely through the spiritual planes that govern the material. It veers all over the mental plane, blaming others for the destruction it causes on the physical level!

How do you begin to train such a confused mind? *Meditation.* There are many levels to this spiritual practice, but the first training is to get the mind to focus on one beautiful thought and to remain there for a good duration. This practice deepens organically as you continue to sit for longer periods.

Change the way your mind thinks by rewiring the neural pathways in your brain. Positive affirmations and power statements, coupled with visualisation, are sure techniques to alter the way your mind works. Ultimately, in each moment, decide that the motivation of thought must come from the higher realms of Spirit.

Power Focus
Reject suggestions of your mind that you have difficulties which make triumph impossible. Cleanse each negative thought as it surfaces with thoughts of Love. Answer your mind with the sweetness of your Soul.

Power Statement
"God's Mind and my mind are one and the same."

You bring blessings of Spirit to
yourself and others through your
spoken or silent word.

Your Spoken Word – The Power to Create

God's gift to you is Power. Power to create heaven on earth; Power to bring beauty to every direction your holy eye sees; Power to transmute all suffering into sweet blossoms in the Garden of Love. It is the power and dominion over your mind, your body, and your life.

All unhappiness arises from lack of power. When you imagine you are weak, and a victim of circumstances over which you have no control, you negate the Divine Power in you. In that moment, you deny the God in you. *Any denial of Spirit causes pain, discomfort and discord in your being, because you are cosmically designed to be in Spirit, every hour, every minute and every second of every day!* Look around the sea of human existence with spiritual vision, and you will see that the prevalence of stress, hardship and disharmony is due to the lack of awareness of Infinite Intelligence.

One of the ways you use this power is through the words you speak. Your spoken words are your verbalised thoughts. They reflect your beliefs, your attitude and your emotions, and all of them have a *creative binding force* that shapes your reality. They each vibrate at specific frequencies, depending on the nature of your thought. And each frequency has attractor patterns which magnetises more of the same frequency to itself! Can you see how a spoken word is not just a word that has nothing to do with your experience and the creation of your life? You, as a divine being, constantly call your experiences to you through your speech.

As Spirit in a human form, your words are the creative expression of your Light, your Beauty and your Grace. Behind the sounds are the living currents of truth that radiate from your consciousness and Spirit. These living currents of truth heal as they expand the power of Love into the thought fields of this world. Words are simply their symbolic representatives. You can speak the word of healing if you so choose. To activate the full power of the healing, you simply have to believe the certainty of this miracle.

Your words sculpt and mould sound and light into bright forms or cast shadows across the landscape of your experience. Observe your speech. Do the words express happiness and delight which means you will attract more of that? Or do they convey lack, limitation and fear which you will get more of, even though it is not what you want on a conscious level? Words are the creative expression of your Spirit. Use them wisely and with joy.

Power Focus

Endeavour to speak consciously and with precision. Such impeccability is the hallmark of an awakened soul.

Power Statement

"My spoken Word carries the power of Spirit."

Your personal life is the mirror of your Supreme Self. If the reflection is distorted, it's a Divine Invitation for you to do the blessed work on yourself.

Your Personal Life – Mirror of Your Soul

As you step forth into the noble Spirit of who you are, more of your spiritual gifts and talents will be revealed. There is more Power available for the awakened Soul to assist in the Great Transition taking place on a planetary and universal level. Living information floods into earth's biosphere from the far end of the Universe at every pulse. To access this alchemical Knowledge, every domain of your physical life has to be aligned to Spirit, where Love and Light rules the order of the day. Transformation must be comprehensive for your authentic Spirit to be fully grounded in matter.

Your personal life is the clear mirror that shows you where your work is still being undone. It indicates where illusion is still masking the truth of who you are from your awareness.

How do you get on with each member of your human family? Irritation indicates there is still error in your perception. Your judgement is in the way. Blame indicates a deep-seated belief of victimhood in a subtle form. It's your refusal to claim self-responsibility for co-creating the relationship as it is. Disappointment shows the lack of true acceptance, of seeing the soul exactly where he or she is in the evolutionary journey.

There are spiritual gifts and blessings behind every conflict. Each becomes a miracle to hasten you Home to your Love, the Spirit of who you truly are. Healing these relationships is to be whole again.

If you can't bring about change in your own life, how can you bring the necessary change on a global and planetary front? If you can't restore harmony quickly in your own heart, how can you heal another's conflict in their psyche or soul?

To bridge the illusion of separation with the immediate people around you is to close the chasm between humanity itself. Everyone needs to make this quantum leap into the new paradigm of Spirit.

Deepen your wider understanding through sorting out the nitty-gritty aspects of your personal life. Do not hide behind the activity of cosmic work, the identity of being a therapist, a healer, a Light Worker and still scowl at your loved ones at home. The heart must stay open 24/7 for your Divine Spirit to reside in. Use this mirror to see your Soul.

You have the Divine Power to make all relationships anew. Believe in this Power. All human clashes are indicative that the personality, and not your Spirit, is hooking up in the interaction. Love is greater than your critical mind.

Power Focus

With families, see your kinship beyond this lifetime. See the bond of Love and nothing else.

Power Statement

"I choose to disengage from old emotional patterns and interact on the higher level as Spirit."

Let your work and the Love of what you are, be one and the same.

Your Work – Your Perfect Self-Expression

As humans rapidly enter a new field of consciousness in alignment with its cosmic destiny, the ethics and values placed upon their work life will change forever. At the moment, the way things are at the workplace does not serve you on the highest level.

The split between your Spirit Self and your matter-based identity has caused you to fragment. You wear different faces at different places, and no longer move forward to greet each moment as your whole self. Each side of life gets to see an incomplete portion of you. You hide away certain aspects, so your full shining countenance is never seen by the people in your work life. You remain a jigsaw with other parts of you omitted from the whole picture of your grand Self. This is so because you have a belief that it is not possible for you to be who you really are and still fit into the work paradigm.

Why do you work? What is the true reason that you give up so many earthly hours of your precious time, to languish in an environment that requires you to keep the Spirit of who you are under wraps? Is this really required, or is it a cultural belief you have unwittingly adopted?

Some work for physical reasons. They trade their passion, their vitality, their dreams, in exchange for bits of paper and metal to provide for the body. Some work for emotional reasons. They use the work place as an arena to play out their emotional patterns. They get their highs and lows from it. Then there are those who enjoy the mental stimulation they get for their intellect to be challenged.

Now, with the mass awakening of the Love Spirit in humankind, there is a fresh breed of individuals who have moved into the new frontier of human existence. By being their authentic Self, the Great Work of Divine Plan is being carried out. They don't wait for the world to change. Instead, they *become the change* for the world. Their perspective towards the human race is a kind and loving one. They move and flow to the rhythm of an all inclusive Intelligence that contains the entire fabric of life. No one is excluded from their Love. They are very excited to be here at such an unprecedented time in human history to assist in this planetary shift. You too are amongst these holy ones.

You are slowly awakening to the truth that work is Love made visible. Be a clear channel of Spirit in your workplace. Whatever your daily job may entail, the greatest gift you have is to be the impeccable Love that you are. Work will no longer be the toil of flesh, but the perfect expression of the Highest in you. When there is a wedge between what you are, and the person you are at work, your soul suffers. Your human system will break down. How can you best serve you and Life through your work? Bring Light into your work. Bring Love into your work. This is your perfect self-expression and service to humanity.

Power Focus
View what you do as an intrinsic part of what you are – a Being of Light. Don't hold back your Love.

Power Statement
"My work is the perfect expression of my Love."

Time is the doorway of Light with which your God Self enters into the physical dimension.

Time – The Everlasting Moment

Time is an earthly construct, a container. It sequences your life events into morning, noon and night; youth, middle years and old age; past, present and future. It splits who you are into chronological proceedings which divide you into three meaningless parts. This learned behaviour of human living is obsolete in the piercing presence of Now. The truth is that you are reborn each time you allow a glorious new belief to enter. All you have been before no longer stays the same, but shifts, moves and reorganises itself to allow for the infusion of the new in you. Just like the flowing river, it's never the same each time you look at it.

When consciousness constricts its own expansive nature, it becomes mind and clings to Time. So while the human eye sees Time as something outside itself, in essence, Time is Consciousness, Time is Being, Time is You, disguised as doing.

Time itself has nothing to do with agendas, schedules, clocks and calendars. When you associate Time to be something that you have to abide by in order to fulfil all the things you have to do, you are caught in the illusion of Time. In that instance, you are no longer a human being but a human doing, a prevalent disorder of the modern culture. Racing against the clock becomes the insane expression of who you are. Too many things to do and not enough time to do them becomes the curse of your existence.

Are you trying to get somewhere other than where you are? Are you trying to be something other than what you are? Are your goals a means to an end, because where you are right now is unacceptable?

The true purpose of Time is the enjoyment of the Spirit of who you are. When you break away from the mind's translation of time, STOP, and behold the sweet sound of rain dancing against the window pane. You will feel its aliveness penetrating your soul. Magic appears.

Time is nothing but windows for you to live. To give of your shining Spirit fully and create a trail of beauty and grace behind you when you leave.

Time is not the circle sliced up in twelve segments. That is man-made for the convenience of the human structure on this material realm. Although it has its practical purpose, its true jewel is the offering of a sacred moment for the Love in you to come alive.

Break the spell of artificial time and you will find Time is but a continuous stream of consciousness of your ever Present Self. There is only you experiencing Now, conscious or unconscious of your Infinite Nature. However, when you are conscious as Spirit, the Now moment becomes the bountiful Universe for you to pull into manifestation every delight that takes your fancy. After all, you can only create from the present moment, because the past is a ghost in your memory box, and the future has yet to take its first breath.

Power Focus
Change your relationship with Time. Break free from its tyranny over your existence. See Time as an ever present moment for the God in you to frolic with creation.

Power Statement
"My power to create and access infinite potential lies in the Now."

Your Unknown is about to be made known. You will come to see there is nothing unfriendly about it.

Quantum Awakening – 2012 and Beyond

For the first time in human history, an immense shift is taking place. This important occasion is not only for humankind, but also for the rest of the universe. Terrestrial and extra-terrestrial connections will be enhanced. Communication between the species will be on a more conscious level than it is now for humans.

For the human story, it's a shift from victimhood to self-empowerment. It's a shift from the imprisoning clutches of fear, to the sweet open arms of Love. It is the ultimate shift from programmed humanness to natural Divinity. This grand miracle is waiting to be fully manifested in you.

These changes have already been taking place, especially on the inner planes for a long time. The consciousness of humanity has been prepared by Infinite

Intelligence, and all its Agents, to such an evolved state that you are all set for the full descent of Spirit. You are ready to walk upon this earth as a God Being and bless all life with your Presence.

Everything on the planet's biosphere will be affected in some way. Change will occur rapidly, rippling across the earth's surface like a gigantic wave. Economic systems based on fear and greed will collapse. Governments and regimes who lack vision of Love and Compassion, whose time in power is more for their own personal gain rather than the progress of its citizens, will be disassembled by its own people.

On a personal level, families that lack true partnership and cohesion will fall apart at the domestic seams. Health scares, breakdown of relationships and insecurity will dominate the private domain. Individuals will have drastic career changes, finally having the courage to follow the calling of their heart.

These are positive changes. It's the emergence of Truth, God's values, and the creative power of Spirit. Unlike the dramatisation of the end of the world in movies, it is simply the end of the world as you know it. *The end of senseless bloodshed, unnecessary starvation, exploitation, and needless suffering.*

Old values based on fear and separation will gradually be a distant memory.

The Mayan, the Hopi, and the Vedic teachings are amongst the many sacred texts that speak about the end of this era of fear ruling the consciousness of mankind. It will be an epoch of hope and optimism, of the constant demonstration of the power of Love, and the might of Spirit. Illusion will not completely disappear, but it will not be regarded as the norm anymore. What was once regarded as sensible and wise will be shown in their true light as foolish and ignorant ways.

This quantum awakening is happening for all. You are now called to align to your spiritual nature. You must orientate your consciousness from matter to Spirit, the true essence of your being. Begin your co-partnership with God now.

Power Focus

Begin to think outside the human stratum. Open your mind to your multidimensional heritage. Much of your cosmic work awaits you.

Power Statement

"I am now ready to embrace my multidimensionality."

*Each one of you who becomes a clear
Love channel for God's Truth will
offset a thousand beings still swayed
by the illusion of fear.*

Your Spiritual Destiny

Your spiritual destiny is to help prepare humanity for this mass awakening. This quantum shift is not just on a global scale, but on a galactic magnitude too. As such, assistance will also be coming from different corners of the galaxies and beyond. Those whose minds are able to de-polarise from matter consciousness, and whose higher intelligence is sufficiently developed, will be able to access this living information of Light and Truth from their starry counterparts.

To carry out the purpose for which you have been born, it is imperative that the paradigm from which you direct and live your life shifts from fear to Love. All aspects of your life have to converge like the spokes of a wheel in the central hub of Spirit. Your relationship with self, with others, your work, including your relationship with God, has to be updated from old modes of existence. Love shall be your motivation, your Power and your currency for everything you require. Elevate your life from senseless routines, unconscious patterns, defensiveness, boredom, negative habits and fear. Follow internal guidance. Tap into your full potential and break out from mediocrity.

What is your higher vision for the world and its people? What is your active contribution to improve things and evolve the understanding of your larger human family? What are your gifts and talents? How are you using them to assist in this planetary shift? These are pertinent questions you must ask yourself on a *daily* basis. This is your final call to fulfil your Spiritual Destiny, to be at the frontier of this cosmic alignment.

Power Focus
Stay conscious in Love to ensure that fear does not motivate you from the subconscious mind. Your focus is to fully fuse the Spirit of God inside you in Matter.

Power Statement
"I am now ready to co-create and be in partnership with Infinite Intelligence."

The simple truth is...
you are here this time round
to be different.

The simple truth is...
you are the creator and creation
in the same moment.

The simple truth is...
you simply are.

About The Author

Ocean WhiteHawk is one of the most dynamic teachers in the field of consciousness and spiritual intelligence today. She is known for her warmth, uncompromising tone and genuine care. Over the last 30 years, Ocean has become highly trained in many areas of personal development, spiritual studies, and metaphysics, and remains at the cutting edge of our soul evolutionary process. Her work is deeply transformational and radical.

She is the author of *JuicyWoman – A Spiritual Guide to Your Feminine Radiance*, a revolutionary book for women of the new millennium. She lives in England, and dedicates her love and passion to awakening souls to the magnificent Truth within them.

Visit www.oceanwhitehawk.com

and change your life

- *Learn more about Ocean's weekly teachings of 'A Course in Miracles' and meditation*

- *Find out about The Enlightened Woman Summits, teaching the power of the Feminine*

- *Discover one-to-one Spiritual Intelligence Mentoring with Ocean*

- *Register for Ocean's 'Provocative Thought of the Week'*

- *Order Ocean's books, audiobooks and CDs*

- *Book Ocean to run seminars in your area or for speaking events*

- *See Ocean's schedule of events*